METAB
DIE

MW01127360

Unlock your body's fat-burning potential with an 8-week Healthy Meal Plan! This guide features delicious recipes for weight loss, muscle building, and getting in shape.

Vincent John Walker

DISCLAIMER

This publication is designed to provide competent and reliable information regarding the subject covered. However, the views expressed in this publication are those of the author alone, and should not be taken as expert instruction or professional advice. The reader is responsible for his or her actions. The author hereby disclaims any responsibility or liability whatsoever that is incurred from the use or application of the contents of this publication by the purchaser of the reader. The purchaser or reader is hereby responsible for his or her actions.

Table of Contents

INTRODUCTION

Accepting the Metabolic Confusion's Power

Metabolic confusion is a beacon of hope and practicality in a world full of fad diets and passing health fads. Welcome to an investigation that will change the way you think about metabolism, nutrition, and the enormous influence these factors have on your life. The "Metabolic Confusion Meal Plan" is a life-changing journey that will help you become a healthier, more energetic version of yourself.

Unraiding the Metabolic Confusion Code

Sometimes it seems like a mystery how our metabolism, that complex symphony of molecular processes coordinating energy usage, works. However, buried deep within this intricacy is a secret that can help us realize our full potential for wellness, including managing our weight. With extensive study and a thorough understanding of human physiology, metabolic confusion emerges as a ground-breaking idea.

Metabolic confusion recognizes our bodies' amazing adaptability. Our bodies may get habituated to regular patterns of calorie consumption and nutrient distribution over time, which can halt weight reduction and health advancement. Through deliberate disruption of these patterns with a well-designed food plan, we may reawaken our metabolism from dormancy, restoring its effectiveness and reaching previously unattainable goals.

Metamorphosis via Dietary Approach

The Metabolic Confusion Meal Plan is an adventure toward overall health, not just a diet. Imagine yourself as full of energy, intelligence, and confidence as you go about your everyday business. Imagine developing a more positive relationship with food, where intentional eating takes the place of impulsive eating and every mouthful brings happiness. Imagine a long-term weight-management strategy that is based on nutrition rather than deprivation.

This meal plan is a customized transformational journey based on your individuality. It embraces uniqueness and acknowledges the fallacy of a one-size-fits-all solution. Rather, it gives you the ability to customize your path so that it fits your unique metabolism, tastes, and way of life.

Using Your Roadmap for Transformation

As you turn the pages that lie ahead, be ready to go on a voyage of comprehension. Explore the science behind metabolic confusion and learn about the complex hormonal and biochemical mechanisms that control your body's response to food. Discover the foundation of a well-balanced diet and learn how to prepare meals that will maintain and enhance your energy metabolism.

Equipped with a thorough plan, you will adopt rotation as the Metabolic Confusion Meal Plan's core tactic. Learn how to intentionally cycle your intake of calories and nutrients to keep your metabolism from becoming too comfortable. With the help of mouthwatering recipes and thorough meal plans, you'll explore weeks full of variety and plenty.

But the trip doesn't end at the dinner table. Learn how the workout and the diet work together to accelerate your progress and improve your overall health. Discover how to overcome challenges, handle social situations with grace, and maintain your accomplishments beyond the early stages.

The Journey of Your Transformation Begins

As the pages turn, keep in mind that you are not just following a diet; rather, you are setting out on a journey that will change your life. Accept the power of metabolic confusion as a tool to transform your physical and mental well-being. Prepare to see the shift that occurs when you honor the complexities of your body, give it purposeful nourishment, and bring its dormant potential to life.

Are you ready to reinvent your story and go on an adventure that brings soul and science together? Now is the time to embark on your transformative journey with the Metabolic Confusion Meal Plan.

THE SCIENCE OF METABOLIC PERPLEXITY

Solving the Mysteries of Metabolism

Few topics in the complex field of human physiology are as fascinating and mysterious as metabolism. It is the complex system that controls how energy is used by our bodies, impacting our weight, energy levels, and general well-being. This chapter takes us on an exploration of the mechanisms, complexities, and multitude of variables that play a part in this fascinating biochemical ballet, intending to demystify metabolism's workings.

A Symphony of Biological Processes: Metabolism

Fundamentally, metabolism is the complex web of chemical processes that keeps us alive. These processes aid in cellular functions, repair, and adaptation by dissolving nutrients and turning them into energy. But the narrative goes much beyond simple energy exchange. It interacts with hormones, genetics, and environmental factors to produce a complex web of interrelated physiological processes.

Understanding the Energy Equation

The basic idea of energy balance is encapsulated in the proverb "calories in, calories out." However, under all of this simplicity is a complex world of dynamics. We will explore the impact of physical activity, the basal metabolic rate, and the thermic effect of food. By looking at weight management through this lens, we will be able to comprehend why it's a multifaceted process that involves complex metabolic reactions rather than just math calculations.

Hormonal Coordination's Elegance

Hormones that control the rate and intensity of different metabolic processes orchestrate metabolism; it is not a solo act. We will explore the complex hormonal landscape that defines our bodies' energy dynamics, from the function of insulin in controlling glucose to the impact of thyroid hormones on the basal metabolic rate. This complex hormonal dance provides fresh insight into how our bodies adjust to different dietary and environmental cues.

Beyond Genes: The Distinctive Metabolism Tapestry

The story of metabolism is personalized by our genetic composition. Our genes influence how our bodies metabolize food, react to physical activity, and even store fat. But genetics is but one paintbrush on this intricate canvas. Changes in lifestyle, sleep habits, stress levels, and the passage of time all interact to affect how quickly metabolism rises and falls. Untangling these variables helps us understand the complex fabric that defines each person's unique metabolic traits.

Introducing the Unveiled—and There's Still More to Learn

We recognize that while we have uncovered many pieces of this complex puzzle, the picture is still incomplete as we navigate the complex terrain of metabolism. This chapter provides the foundational knowledge required to appreciate the severity of metabolic confusion. Equipped with this fundamental understanding, we are prepared to investigate how a carefully designed meal plan can bring about change, awaken latent metabolic potentials, and lead us on the transformative path toward overall well-being.

The Function of Hormones in the Regulation of Metabolism

Hormones: Metabolic Harmony Conductors

Hormones play a central role in the complex realm of metabolic regulation by coordinating a well-balanced group of biochemical reactions that direct our body's use of energy and homeostasis. These chemical messengers have a substantial impact on a variety of physiological processes, including signals of hunger and fullness as well as energy expenditure and storage. This chapter explores the essential hormones that act as cornerstones in the regulation of metabolism, revealing their complex interplay and significant influence.

Insulin: Keeper of the Glucose Equilibrium

Insulin is the primary hormone that regulates metabolism and is produced by the pancreas. Its main function is to regulate blood sugar levels. Insulin helps move glucose from the bloodstream into cells after a carbohydrate meal so that it can be stored as glycogen or used as fuel. Insulin also regulates fat metabolism by preventing fat that has been stored from breaking down. Insulin plays a critical role in maintaining metabolic stability as disorders such as diabetes and metabolic syndrome can result from an imbalance in the hormone's balance.

Glucagon: Activating Stores of Energy

Similar to insulin, glucagon is the opposite. Glucagon, which is secreted by the pancreas, promotes the breakdown of glycogen into glucose and the release of glucose into the blood. It ensures that the body has a constant supply of energy during fasting or low blood sugar episodes. Insulin and glucagon dance together to control blood sugar levels and keep the metabolism in balance.

Leptin: Fulfilling the Hunger

Often referred to as the "satiety hormone," leptin is produced by fat cells and functions as a mediator between the brain and adipose tissue. It has a significant impact on energy balance and appetite control. Leptin levels rise when fat reserves increase, informing the brain that the body has enough energy reserves. On the other hand, persistent overindulgence may result in leptin resistance, which impairs the body's ability to detect energy status correctly and fuels obesity.

Ghrelin: Activating Appetite

The "hunger hormone," ghrelin, emerges from the stomach and counterbalances leptin. Its levels rise before meals and fall afterward. This hormone promotes eating by igniting feelings of hunger. Ghrelin and leptin's complex interactions regulate hunger and satisfaction, influencing our eating habits and promoting metabolic balance.

Thyroid Hormones: Keepers of the Metabolic Pace

Thyroid hormones, which include triiodothyronine (T3) and thyroxine (T4), are produced by the thyroid gland and play a major part in controlling metabolism. They control the body's resting metabolic rate or the amount of energy used, and they have an impact on many other physiological processes, such as digestion and heart rate. Thyroid hormone fluctuations are crucial for maintaining metabolic symmetry since they may cause metabolic abnormalities.

Cortisol: Reacting to Tension

The adrenal glands release cortisol, sometimes known as the "stress hormone," in response to stressful situations. Although its main function is to prepare the body for the "fight or flight" response, long-term stress may result in persistently high cortisol levels. This may interfere with metabolic functions, encouraging the buildup of fat and affecting food preferences. Understanding the effects of cortisol on metabolism reveals the complex relationship between hormones, stress, and overall metabolic health.

The Melodic Ensemble

Just a small portion of the complex hormonal mosaic that controls our metabolism is comprised of these hormones. Their interaction goes beyond single roles to create a well-balanced symphony that reacts to stimuli from the outside world, physical exercise, and nutrition. Understanding their functions and interactions helps us to understand the delicate balance necessary for the best possible metabolic control. As we continue our investigation, we unravel how a well-planned diet may direct and affect this hormonal symphony, leading to life-changing outcomes.

The Advantages of Metabolic Confusion in Managing Weight

Accepting the Benefits of Metabolic Confusion to Manage Weight Effectively

Conventional weight management techniques frequently face a significant obstacle in the form of the body's adaptability. As the body becomes used to regular calorie patterns, diets may cause plateaus and declining results. Step in metabolic confusion, a ground-breaking tactic that upends consistency and rekindles hope for long-term weight reduction. We explore the many benefits of metabolic confusion for weight control in this chapter, providing insight into how this strategy might transform your path to better health.

Overcoming Plateaus with Dynamic Modification

Variability is key to metabolic confusion; it's the art of keeping your body guessing. Through continuous adjustments to calorie intake and nutritional ratios, this method keeps your metabolism from stabilizing at a comfortable pace. This dynamic approach prevents your body from adapting by keeping it on its toes. Consequently, this aids in overcoming weight loss plateaus, which are a typical barrier in conventional diets. Your metabolism stays flexible while you go through stages of different calorie intake, which maximizes its ability to burn calories and helps you lose weight.

Getting the Metabolic Furnace Started

Its capacity to increase your basal metabolic rate (BMR), or the amount of energy used by your body when at rest, is a basic component of metabolic confusion. The deliberate changes in calorie intake force your body to work harder to process food and adjust to shifting nutrient ratios. By keeping the metabolic furnace fired up, calories are burned both when you're moving and when you're at rest. As a result, your body becomes a more effective calorie-burning machine, which promotes long-term, sustainable weight loss.

Protecting Your Lean Muscle Mass

Lean muscular mass is often lost while following traditional restricted diets. On the other hand, muscular tissue maintenance takes precedence in metabolic confusion. When combined with the

15

right amount of protein, the rotation-based method gives your muscles the nutrition they need to grow and thrive. Because muscle tissue needs more energy to maintain than fat tissue, this preservation is essential for preserving a higher basal metabolic rate. Maintaining lean muscle increases your body's ability to burn calories, which will help you lose weight even more.

Refuting Metabolic Adjustment

A typical problem with conventional diets is a metabolic adaptation when the body's reaction to extended calorie restriction prevents further weight reduction. Metabolic confusion cleverly avoids this obstacle. By continuously modifying the amount of calories and nutrients you consume, you prevent your metabolism from slowing down and adjusting to low energy levels. This calculated variance ensures that your weight loss journey stays fruitful and long-lasting by preventing your metabolic rate from plummeting.

Developing Intentional Eating Practices

Metabolic confusion promotes eating with awareness and consciousness. You learn to recognize and understand your body's signals of hunger, fullness, and satisfaction as you progress through different stages of calorie consumption. Your ability to make educated food decisions, give priority to nutrient-rich options, and cultivate a positive relationship with food is enhanced by this increased awareness. This shift from strict dieting to intuitive eating promotes overall wellbeing and long-term success.

A Way Forward for Durable Change

Metabolic confusion goes beyond band-aid fixes and provides a whole approach that takes advantage of your body's unique characteristics to bring about long-term transformation. You can create a path to long-term weight management by embracing variability, increasing your metabolism, protecting muscle mass, resisting adaptation, and encouraging mindful eating. You'll discover this approach's transforming power as you work through its subtleties—not only for changing the way your body looks, but also for changing the way you think about nutrition, health, and overall wellbeing.

GETTING READY FOR ACHIEVEMENT

Evaluating Your Present Consumption Habits

- ***Examining Your Present Consumption Patterns: Crucial Measures and Methods:*** Setting off on a path to better health and nutrition requires a candid assessment of your current eating habits. This crucial stage creates a foundational knowledge of your food choices, preferences, and possible improvement areas. We explore the essential steps and techniques in this part to help you get a complete picture of your current eating patterns.

- ***Keeping a Food Journal: Tracking Your Consumption:*** Maintaining a food diary provides a trustworthy window into what you eat every day. Keep track of all the meals, snacks, and drinks you have throughout the day. Make a note of the ingredients, serving quantities, and any pertinent cooking instructions. This written report reveals patterns such as chronic nutritional imbalances, overindulgence in calories, or insufficient diversity. Patterns will show up over a few days or weeks to help direct changes toward a healthier diet.

- ***Analysis of Nutrients: Revealing Nutritional Value:*** Assessing the amount of nutrients you consume is essential for determining shortages and imbalances. Make use of applications and web resources to examine the nutrients in your food. Pay attention to both important micronutrients and critical macronutrients (fats, proteins, and carbs) (vitamins and minerals). By comparing your consumption with the suggested daily amounts, you may identify any possible problem areas.

- *Meal Schedule and Frequency: Identifying Trends:* Analyze the frequency and timing of your meals. Do you eat at the same times every day or do you often miss meals? Do you see any trends in your impulsive snacking? Identifying periods of overindulgence or irregular eating patterns might help you make the required changes. Regular eating at regular times gives you a consistent supply of energy and helps control your metabolism and appetite.

- *Diversity and Equilibrium: Assessing the Variety of Foods:* Analyze the variety and harmony of your food. Is there a variety of vibrant fruits and veggies, lean meats, complete grains, and healthy fats on your plate? A diet rich in a variety of foods provides a greater variety of nutrients that are essential for good health. Look for methods to add more diversity if you notice a shortage of certain meal categories or monotony.

- *Controlled Portioning: Importance of Serving Sizes:* Calorie intake is significantly influenced by portion size. Determine how big your servings are and contrast them with the suggested serving sizes. Overindulgence may result in an excessive intake of calories, even when it involves nutrient-dense meals. Unintentional calorie excess may be avoided by engaging in mindful eating practices and paying attention to portion sizes.

- *Recognizing Your Emotional and Mindful Food Triggers:* Consider your inclinations toward mindful and emotional eating. Do you often turn to food as a coping mechanism or when you're stressed? Understanding the emotions that lead to overeating gives insight into situations when better coping mechanisms may be used.

- *Hydration Procedures: Monitoring Fluid Consumption:* Never undervalue the significance of maintaining proper hydration. Sufficient hydration is essential for general health. Make a note of how much water, herbal teas, and other liquids you consume each day. Make sure you're getting the amount of water your body needs.

- *Culinary Techniques: Styles of Cooking and Preparation:* Evaluate your cooking techniques. Do you cook at home or do you eat a lot of takeout and prepared foods? Meals prepared at home often provide you with more control over the materials and serving amounts. Assess your cooking methods as well; choosing to sauté, steam, or grill instead of deep fry may make a big difference in the nutritional value of your food.

- *Self-Examination: Individual Assessment:* Consider your eating habits with reflection. Think about how you feel about food, what makes you choose unhealthy options, how you handle urges, and how you feel about eating in general. This self-assessment helps you get a better understanding of your driving forces and possible obstacles to changing for the better.

When you systematically use these techniques to evaluate your current eating patterns, you create the foundation for wise choices and positive changes that support your goals for health and well-being.

Having Reasonable Expectations and Goals

A solid foundation of reasonable expectations and goals is necessary before embarking on a journey to achieve your health and fitness objectives. You may prevent disappointment and put yourself in a position for long-term success by setting realistic objectives and seeing your path ahead. In this comprehensive video, we go through the process of setting reasonable goals and expectations step-by-step.

- *Introspection and Assessment:* Before setting goals, evaluate your current level of general well-being, fitness, and health. Take into account your skills, constraints, way of life, and prior goal-setting encounters. Accept your achievements as well as your areas for improvement. This self-examination provides a strong basis for creating your goals.

- *Set Particular Objectives:* Establish quantifiable, clear goals that align with your objectives. Set measurable objectives like "run a 5K event within six weeks" or "drop 10 pounds in three months" instead of vague ones like "get in shape" or "reduce weight." This precision will help you track your progress and measure your success.

- *Set quantifiable goals for yourself.* Give your goals numerical measurements or metrics. Having concrete metrics, such as pounds lost, inches lowered, or kilometers run, enables you to track your progress efficiently. This information is essential for planning your journey and making any necessary adjustments along the way.

- *Realistic and Achievable Objectives:* Make sure the goals you have set are sensible and attainable. Desperation and discontent may result from setting unrealistic goals. Consider your current financial situation, responsibilities, and lifestyle. For instance, it may not be possible to plan to work out seven days a week if your calendar is too busy. Adapt your goals to the circumstances you find yourself in.

- *In Line with Your Priorities and Values:* Your priorities and values should align with your goals. Think about the reasons these goals are significant to you. Making the connection between your objectives and your underlying motivations increases your commitment and tenacity. Knowing that getting better cardiovascular health would free up more time for you to spend with your kids or go on outdoor activities will inspire you to take action.

- *Appropriate Deadlines:* Decide on deadlines for completing your goals. This dissuades procrastination and fosters a feeling of urgency. A deadline drives consistent effort; try aiming for "exercise for 30 minutes, four times a week, over the next three months" instead of "exercise more."

- *Divide Up Larger Goals:* If your ultimate goal is big, break it up into smaller, more manageable tasks. This makes your journey easier and makes you feel accomplished as you go. If your ultimate goal is to run a marathon, for instance, start with smaller goals like a 5K and work your way up to longer distances.

- *Flexibility and adaptability:* Life is not static; things may change. Be ready to adjust your objectives in the event of unforeseen issues, disappointments, or reordering of priorities. Being adaptable helps people feel less hopeless when things don't go as planned. The mark of resilience is adaptation, not failure.

- *Track Development and Honor Significant Occasions:* Maintain a frequent progress log and acknowledge your achievements, no matter how little they may seem. Milestone celebrations encourage good conduct and boost motivation. It acts as a reminder that despite your sluggish growth, you are still making progress.

- **Gain from Difficulties:** Anticipate challenges on the journey. View obstacles as opportunities for advancement rather than as barriers. Take lessons from failures, analyze the reasons behind them, and modify your approach appropriately. Taking the initiative increases your ability to overcome challenges.

- **Have perseverance and patience:** Finally, remember that patience is required to achieve long-term results. Perseverance and patience are essential traits. Pay more attention to the procedure than the finished result. One significant aspect of the shift is travel.

Establishing a Helpful Setting for Your Trip

Setting out on a path to improve your health and wellbeing is greatly impacted by the environment you cultivate. Creating an atmosphere that is encouraging may spur achievement and increase the accessibility and sustainability of healthy choices. We'll dive into doable strategies in this book to create a space that empowers and elevates your journey.

- **Get Rid of the Clutter:** To reduce noise and promote calmness, tidy up your physical area. Having your surroundings well-organized might help you think more clearly and make healthier judgments.

24

- ***Stock Up on Nutrient-Rich Foods:*** Stow a variety of nutrient-dense, healthy foods in your refrigerator and pantry. Keep an assortment of healthful grains, lean meats, fresh produce, and healthy fats in your diet. This makes it so that making healthy decisions comes naturally to you.

- ***Plan Your Meals and Snacks:*** Make a list of the meals and snacks you will eat. Make a weekly meal plan and prep the items ahead of time to prevent rushed, unhealthy decisions.

- ***Establish a Workout Zone:*** Set aside a space at home just for exercise. Whether it's a weight room, an exercise mat, or a yoga nook, having a dedicated area promotes consistent activity.

- ***Establish Visible Inspirations:*** Put visual cues about your objectives in key places. Put your written goals, motivational sayings, or inspirational pictures somewhere you'll see them often, like the bathroom mirror or refrigerator.

- ***Embrace a Positive Environment:*** Create a happy vibe by surrounding oneself with inspiring people. This might include connecting with encouraging friends and family, reading books that inspire, or listening to podcasts that encourage.

- ***Seek Social Support:*** Make connections with others who have similar health objectives. Participate in local organizations, online forums, or fitness courses to share knowledge, suggestions, and inspiration.

- *Select an Accountability Partner:* Find a companion who is on the same path as you and who can provide encouragement, accountability, and a feeling of duty.

- *Minimize Temptations:* Make fewer unhealthy temptations available to you in your environment. If there are foods that make you feel indulgent, hide them from view to reduce the likelihood of overindulging.

- *Outfit Your Kitchen:* Invest in gadgets that make cooking easier. Superior kitchen tools, organizers, and culinary devices may improve your experience in the kitchen and meal preparation.

- *Make Restful Sleep a Priority:* Establish a setting that encourages restful sleep. Make sure your bedroom is peaceful, well-lit, and distraction-free. Getting enough good sleep is essential for general health.

- *Remain Hydrated:* Always have a water bottle handy, either on your desk or in your hands throughout the day. Your health depends on you being hydrated, and having ready access to water encourages this.

- *Incorporate things that favorably stimulate your senses to enhance your sensory experience.* A harmonious atmosphere may be enhanced by artwork, fragrant candles, fresh flowers, and relaxing music.

- *Detox from Screens:* To promote healthy behaviors, set limitations on screen usage and think about designating certain hours as screen-free times.

- *Develop a Regular Self-Care Routine:* Set aside time for self-care exercises that encourage calmness and stress reduction. Spending time outside, taking a long bath, or practicing meditation all help to create a loving atmosphere.

- *Celebrate Your Success:* Put medals from races or a graphic depicting your advancement on display as reminders of your triumphs. They act as a continual reminder of your accomplishments.

- *Periodically Assess and Adjust:* Keep an eye on how your surroundings are affecting your travels. Determine which areas want improvement, then make the necessary adjustments.

THE METABOLIC CONFUSION MEAL PLAN'S BASIS

Macronutrients: An Unveiling

- ***Revealing the Nature of Macronutrients: Comprehending the Fundamental Components of Diet:*** The idea of macronutrients, or the basic components that influence our food choices, is at the core of nutritional research. Made up of lipids, proteins, and carbs, these vital elements are crucial for supplying our bodies with the energy they need to operate. In this investigation, we peel back the layers of complexity surrounding macronutrients, illuminating their importance and vital functions within the intricate web of nutrition.

- ***Carbohydrates: The Main Source of Energy:*** Our diet is based mostly on carbohydrates, which are sometimes referred to as the body's "preferred" source of energy. Carbohydrates, which are included in meals including grains, fruits, vegetables, and legumes, are converted into glucose, an essential fuel that drives the synthesis of energy inside cells. There are two main types of them: basic and sophisticated. Simple carbs, found in fruit and candy sweets, are rapidly absorbed and provide you with immediate energy boosts. Whole grains and vegetables are rich sources of complex carbs, which release energy more gradually and promote long-term energy.

- **Proteins: The Building Elements of Life:** Amino acids are the fundamental building blocks needed for the synthesis and upkeep of tissues, hormones, enzymes, and a variety of other critical components. Proteins are known as the body's "building blocks." Proteins are found in foods including meats, fish, dairy, legumes, and nuts. They are essential for immune system function, muscle repair, and the creation of important chemicals.

- **Fats: Essential for Essential Activities:** Fats are essential to many body processes and are often seen as both necessary and concerning. Saturated, unsaturated, and trans fats are the body's energy stores; they also protect important organs, make it easier for fat-soluble vitamins to be absorbed, and keep cell membrane integrity intact. Selecting nutritious sources such as avocados, nuts, seeds, and fatty fish provides vital fatty acids that our systems are unable to create on their own, even if moderation is still important.

- **Bringing the Whole Symphony into Harmony: Meeting Specific Needs:** Achieving optimal health requires a careful balance of these macronutrients. There isn't a single strategy that works for everyone, though; the right balance depends on several variables, including age, level of physical activity, metabolism, and personal health goals. Athletes might need to consume more protein, while people trying to lose weight might need to adjust how much carbohydrates they eat. Customizing the macro ratio to each person's needs involves a journey of self-discovery and health optimization.

- ***Wholesome Options Boost Quality Compared to Processed Alternatives:*** Making whole, unprocessed foods a priority in your diet helps you get the most out of your intake of macronutrients. Not only do whole grains, lean proteins, and healthy fats provide a range of additional nutrients, such as fiber, vitamins, and minerals, but they also help create a balanced macro profile. On the other hand, processed foods that are high in added sugars, bad fats, and refined carbohydrates can upset the balance and lead to health problems.

- ***Intelligent Feeding of the Body and Mind through Mindful Nourishment:*** Mindful eating is empowered by an understanding of macronutrients. You can create meals that support your health goals if you recognize their roles. Emphasizing nutrient-dense, unprocessed foods while allowing occasional indulgences strikes a sustainable equilibrium. The trick lies in establishing an approach that nourishes your body, mind, and general well-being.

In the complicated field of nutrition, macronutrients are the building blocks. They guide intelligent food choices, give energy, promote tissue health, and preserve important processes. By recognizing their importance and accepting a well-rounded method, you start on a road of total nutrition and holistic wellbeing.

The Benefits of Balanced Diets

Using Balanced Meals to Their Full Potential: Promoting Health and Energy

- In the ever-changing world of nutrition, balanced meals are essential building blocks for reaching optimum health and wellbeing. These meals carefully combine the three main macronutrients—proteins, fats, and carbohydrates—with a wide range of micronutrients to provide your body with complete sustenance. In this investigation, we explore how balanced meals might improve energy and general wellbeing as well as their transforming potential.

Harmony of Nutrients: A Comprehensive Method

- Well-balanced meals represent a harmonic confluence of nutrients rather than just a mishmash of foods. Fats support cellular processes and nutrition absorption, proteins support muscle development and repair, and carbohydrates provide the energy to power your activities. These macronutrients work together to provide satiety, sustained energy levels, and the prevention of energy crashes.

Normal Blood Sugar: Reliable Energy

- A balanced meal has a significant impact on blood sugar levels. The combination of lipids, proteins, and carbs slows down the pace at which glucose enters the system, preventing sudden increases and decreases in blood sugar. This steady regulation of blood sugar results in energy that lasts the whole day, which promotes increased focus and efficiency.

Improved Absorption of Nutrients and Digestion

- Every macronutrient is essential to the process of digestion. Proteins need certain enzymes to break down, carbohydrates start the digestive process, and fats help the body absorb fat-soluble vitamins and other vital minerals. When you include all three into a meal, you maximize the effectiveness of your body's digestion process, ensuring optimal nutritional absorption.

Controlling Appetite and Satiety

- Well-balanced meals have a significant impact on controlling hunger. Proteins and fats help to avoid overindulgence by promoting feelings of fullness and happiness. This becomes particularly important when trying to control weight since eating balanced meals makes you feel fuller and less likely to overeat or nibble on the spur of the moment.

Promoting the health and healing of muscles

- Balanced meals are essential for maintaining muscular health and promoting post-exercise recovery for those who engage in physical activity. Proteins provide the critical amino acids needed for muscle repair, while carbs help with recovery by replenishing glycogen reserves. Including these nutrients in well-balanced diets promotes optimal physical function and lowers the chance of muscle deterioration.

Fulfilling the Need for Micronutrients

- Macronutrients are just one aspect of a balanced diet; they also act as a vehicle for a variety of vital vitamins and minerals. By consuming a wide variety of colorful fruits and vegetables, whole grains, lean meats, and healthy fats, you are providing your body with the micronutrients it needs to maintain strong bones, a robust immune system, and general wellness.

Creating Holistic Harmony: Promoting Nutritional Health

- Beyond their physiological advantages, well-balanced meals support overall health and wellbeing. A steady intake of nutrition helps to maintain emotional and mental stability. Sufficient consumption of nutrients such as omega-3 fatty acids, which are obtained from fatty fish, supports mental well-being and emotional balance.

Creating Your Equitable Plate: Useful Advice

- A combination of science and creativity is needed to create balanced meals. Aim to load your plate with a variety of nutrient-dense meals, including whole grains like brown rice or quinoa, lean proteins like chicken, fish, or plant-based substitutes, a rainbow of colorful veggies, and healthy fats like nuts, avocados, and olive oil.

Boosting Your Path to Wellbeing

- Despite the prevalence of diet fads and quick solutions, balanced meals continue to be a powerful and time-tested method of taking care of your health. When you embrace the synergy between macronutrients and an abundance of nutrients, you improve your health, energy, and vitality and help to create a life that is full of holistic well-being.

When to Eat to Promote Optimal Metabolism

- ***When to Eat Strategically to Boost Your Metabolism:*** The time of your meals becomes important in the complex dance of nutrition and metabolism because it affects how your body uses nutrients and energy. You may be able to improve your metabolism and general health by aligning your eating habits with your body's natural cycles. This investigation explores the science of meal scheduling to maximize metabolic potential.

- *Accepting Circadian Rhythms: The Internal Clock of Your Body:* Your body runs on a 24-hour cycle of physiological activities coordinated by an internal clock called the circadian rhythm. Hormone release, sleep cycles, metabolism, and other processes are all impacted by this rhythm. You may access your body's innate efficiency by respecting its natural rhythm.

- *Opening the Metabolic Spark for Breakfast:* It is well acknowledged that having a balanced breakfast is essential to starting your day off right. Your body receives this as a signal to begin energy use and metabolic activities. A high-protein breakfast can increase metabolism, reduce appetite, and regulate blood sugar levels.

- *Spaced Meals: Preventing Low Energy:* Instead of treating yourself to large, occasional meals, think about distributing your meals equally. Frequent little meals spaced a few hours apart may help keep blood sugar levels stable and prevent low energy spikes. This steady flow of energy prevents overindulgence and maintains metabolic activity.

- *Pre-Workout Fuel: Get Your Exercise Energized:* Another way to influence metabolism is to time your meals to coincide with your exercise. Eating a healthy lunch or snack before doing out provides your body with energy that is accessible to use right away. Proteins and carbs together may improve performance and speed up muscle repair after exercise.

- **Refueling and Repairing After Exercise:** Your body is more suited to absorb nutrients that aid in muscle repair and recovery after exercise. This process is accelerated by a post-workout meal or snack high in proteins and carbs, which maximizes muscle development and regeneration.

- **Evening Meals: Calm and Reflection:** When the day is coming to an end, choosing nutrient-dense evening meals in moderation may promote improved digestion and quality of sleep. Avoiding large, high-calorie meals just before bed will help prevent upset stomachs and sleep disruptions.

- **Preventing Extended Fasting: Maintaining a Steady Metabolism:** Although there has been some focus on intermittent fasting, prolonged fasting may slow down metabolism and cause energy to be lost. Even during periods of fasting, maintaining a healthy metabolic rate and avoiding muscle breakdown may be achieved by strategically timing your meals.

- **Hydration: A Crucial Timing Component:** It's important to pay attention to when you drink water. Drinking plenty of water is essential for a healthy metabolism. Digestion and nutrient absorption are facilitated by drinking water throughout the day and making sure you're hydrated before meals.

- ***Customization: Sensitive to Your Form:*** Recall that everyone reacts differently to the time of meals. To fine-tune your strategy, pay attention to your body's signs about appetite, energy levels, and performance. Your body often speaks louder than any strict food plan about what it needs.

- ***Finding a Balance: Aligning Meal Schedule with Your Way of Life:*** It is very important to schedule meals according to your lifestyle and tastes. Even while studies suggest that the time of your meals might affect your metabolism, eating a balanced diet generally and consistently forming good habits are still very important. Aim for a diet that is nutrient-rich and well-balanced, and think about experimenting with meal schedules to find what works best for your particular body.

THE STRATEGY OF ROTATION

Recognizing the Macronutrient and Calorie Rotation

Revealing Nutritional Dynamics with Rotation of Calorie and Macronutrients: In the world of nutrition, the idea of rotating macronutrients and calories indicates a strategy that goes beyond fixed eating patterns. By varying your intake of calories and the key macronutrients—carbs, proteins, and fats—you may enhance your metabolism, accelerate your progress, and strengthen your bond with food. This study delves deeply into the intricate physics of rotating calories and macronutrients for a comprehensive understanding.

Rotating Calorie Sources Boosts Metabolic Flexibility: Calorie rotation is the process of switching between intervals of higher and lower calorie intake. This approach aims to prevent the metabolic adaptation that prolonged calorie restriction may cause. By gradually increasing your caloric intake, you may avoid weight loss or muscle-building plateaus and instruct your body to maintain an efficient metabolism.

Rotation of Macronutrients: Variability and Adaptation in Nutrient: The goal of macronutrient rotation is to alter the ratios of carbohydrates, proteins, and fats in your diet. This exercise promotes change and tests your body's ability to adapt. For example, alternating days with high and low carbs may sustain energy requirements while promoting efficient fat use.

A Difference in Macronutrients in Cyclical Ketosis: In cyclical ketosis, carbohydrate intake varies between days with low and high carbohydrate content. A lot of people who follow ketogenic diets use this tactic. In addition to frequently refueling glycogen stores for prolonged energy during strenuous activity or improved thyroid function, it aims to profit from ketosis.

Diverse Cuisines and Intuitive Eating: Establishing a Good Connection with Food: Intuitive eating involves paying attention to your body's signals and consuming food based on feelings of hunger, fullness, and satisfaction. Despite not following a strict rotation of calories or macronutrients, intuitive eating encourages flexibility and lets you enjoy a variety of meals without feeling bad. By using this technique, you may enhance your psychological relationship with food and prevent feelings of deprivation.

Periodization of Fitness: Enhancing Performance: Rotating calories and macronutrients is a common training strategy used by athletes to improve their performance. Periodization is the process of matching food to training stages to guarantee maximum performance, recovery, and energy availability. This might include consuming more carbohydrates during demanding training sessions and altering during periods of rest or recuperation.

Customization Is Essential for Adapting the Strategy: How well each person responds to calorie and macronutrient rotation varies. Objectives, degree of activity, metabolism, and individual preferences are all significant factors. You may get help from a qualified nutritionist or dietitian in creating a rotation plan that meets your needs and objectives.

Practical Application: Organizing and Supervising: When adopting the rotation of macronutrients and calories, planning and monitoring are necessary. You may keep on track by carefully distributing macronutrients and scheduling days with greater and lower consumption. Applications and notebooks for tracking food intake may provide data on trends and advancements.

Variety and Consistency in Balance: A Long-Term Sustainable Strategy: Rotating calories and macronutrients is good, but consistency is key. To be successful over the long run, adherence and variance must be balanced. Regularly assess your body's reactions and adjust as necessary to optimize progress.

Taking Charge of Your Dietary Path: Examining the area of rotating calories and macronutrients adds a dynamic element to your nutritional strategy. By introducing sporadic fluctuations in calories and macronutrients, you test the boundaries of your body's resistance and improve metabolic flexibility. You may get better results, have more energy, and have a lasting relationship with nutrition by customizing this approach to meet your requirements.

Creating Your Custom Rotation Schedule

Creating Your Tailored Rotation Schedule: A Guide to Tailored Diet: When it comes to nutrition, the idea of a customized rotation plan provides a calculated method for making the best nutritional decisions. You may adjust your calorie intake and the macronutrients (fats, proteins, and carbs) you consume to improve your metabolism, reach your health objectives, and develop a long-term eating habit. With the help of this guidance, you may create a rotation schedule that suits your requirements and tastes.

Step 1: Establish Your Objectives and Goals

Start by defining your goals for fitness and wellness. Do you want to lose weight, increase muscle, have more energy, or perform better in sports? Your rotation strategy is constructed on a solid grasp of your objectives.

Step 2: Assess Your Way of Life and Routine

Take into account your exercise levels, daily schedule, and lifestyle requirements. Do you need extra energy on certain days or at certain periods of the day? Do you need to modify your diet during times of rest or recuperation? Adapting your strategy to your way of life will guarantee sustainability and usability.

Step 3: Select Your Rotation Technique

Choose the rotation strategy that best fits your objectives. Do you like to alternate between macronutrients and calories, or maybe both? Select a strategy that suits your needs and is most likely to get the results you are looking for.

Calculate the Rotation Frequency in Step 4

Choose the frequency of calorie and macronutrient rotation. This might include weekly shifts, monthly variances, or even daily alterations. The frequency will vary according to your objectives, the response of your metabolism, and the flexibility of your body.

Step 5: Establish High and Low Goals

Establish the ranges for high and low calorie and macronutrient consumption. You may eat extra calories or adjust your macronutrient ratios on days when you consume more to meet your greater energy demands. You might establish a calorie deficit or concentrate on a different macronutrient distribution on days when you consume less.

Step 6: Record Your Exercise Days

If you exercise often, think about your training plan. To enhance performance and facilitate effective recuperation, it might make sense to schedule higher intake days around periods of intensive activity. Adapt the ratios of your macronutrients to the needs of your exercises.

Step 7: Accept Diversity in Diet

Make sure a variety of nutrient-dense foods are included in your rotation plan. This improves your general well-being and stops your diet from becoming monotonous. Try a variety of food sources to achieve your macronutrient objectives.

Step 8: Give nutrient balance a priority

Maintain a balanced nutritional profile while switching up your macronutrients and calories. Make sure you're getting enough fiber, vitamins, and minerals from a range of sources. Steer clear of drastic adjustments that might cause dietary imbalances.

Step 9: Observe and Modify

Evaluate your progress regularly and note how your body reacts to the rotation plan. Pay attention to shifts in your level of performance, energy, and general well-being. Be ready to modify your plan in light of your observations.

Step 10: Seek Professional Advice

It is advisable to consult a registered dietitian or other nutrition professional if you are unfamiliar with rotation plans or have particular health concerns. They can assist in customizing your plan to meet your needs and provide advice on how to carry it out successfully.

Step 11: Accept Adaptability

Recall that the rotation plan is an ever-changing instrument. Since life is always changing, your dietary requirements may also change. Adopt a flexible mindset and modify your strategy as necessary to continue moving in the direction of your goals.

Boost Your Dietary Adventure

Creating a personalized rotation plan gives you the ability to manage your diet in a manner that fits your objectives and way of life. You may create a more resilient dietary pattern, increased energy levels, and improved metabolic response by carefully alternating your macronutrient and calorie intake. Your rotation plan turns into a dynamic approach that changes as you do as you go toward your ideal state of health and wellbeing.

Modifying the Rotation Approach to Fit Various Lifestyles

Customizing the Rotation Strategy to Various Lifestyles: Providing Flexibility for Everyone

A rotation strategy's flexibility to fit different lifestyles is what makes it so beautiful. The rotation technique may be tailored to your situation, whether you have a demanding work schedule, are a serious athlete, or place a high priority on your family. The rotation technique may be modified as follows to fit various lifestyles:

The Preoccupied Expert

Planning is essential for those with busy job schedules. You may maintain focus on your goals even on busy days by preparing meals or snacks ahead of time. Choose healthy, straightforward solutions that fit into your rotating schedule. Use meal planning strategies to make sure you always have a variety of well-balanced options available.

The Intense Performer

Athletes might alter their rotation plans to help with their training and recovery. Focus on protein and carbs on days when you work out hard to feed your body and help heal your muscles. Try adjusting your plan to align with lower energy use on rest days.

The Butterfly of Socialization:

Eating out and navigating social gatherings might be challenging, but it is possible. Make a plan by looking over choices and selecting options that align with your rotation goals. If you anticipate consuming more calories during social events, be sure to offset that with fewer days before or after the event.

The Individual Focused on Family

Include your family members in your rotation plan if you're juggling family responsibilities. Make wholesome dinners that the whole family will enjoy. Choose adaptable ingredients to accommodate a range of palates while staying within your rotational constraints.

The Passionate Traveler

Your rotation plan doesn't have to be disrupted by travel. Bring wholesome snacks for the journey and look for locations nearby that provide wholesome options. When you return to your routine, try to continue your rotation plan if you run into difficulties while traveling.

The Chef with Intuition

If you eat more intuitively, use the concepts of rotation while paying attention to your body's cues. Make an effort to eat a range of foods high in nutrients, and modify your consumption according to your degree of hunger, fullness, and energy.

The Families Aware of Their Health

A rotation plan may be a cooperative effort for families. Include your family in the planning and preparation of meals. Teach them about the idea of rotation and work together to prepare meals that satisfy everyone's dietary requirements.

The Employee Who Shifts

Because of their erratic schedules, shift workers have particular difficulties. It is necessary to schedule meals and snacks by your shift hours if you decide to modify the rotation plan. To maintain your energy levels, stick to regular meal times and give priority to nutrient-rich selections.

The Long-Range Planner

Try out various rotation frequencies and techniques if you're determined to stick with the rotation approach for the long run. Monitor your development over time and adjust your strategy in response to your body's response.

The Flexible Method

And lastly, flexibility is crucial. Because life is dynamic, things change. As your requirements and objectives change, be open to making adjustments while adhering to your rotation strategy.

RECIPES AND WEEKLY MEAL PLANS FOR THE 8 WEEKS

How to Start the Metabolic Fire in the First Week

Day 1: Exciting Beginning

- Eggs scrambled with spinach and tomatoes for breakfast
- whole-grain toast
- a fresh fruit salad
- Lunch consists of grilled chicken salad dressed with a balsamic vinaigrette, cucumbers, bell peppers, and mixed greens.
- Snack: Berries and Greek yogurt drizzled with honey
- Steamed broccoli and baked salmon served with quinoa for dinner

Day 2: Act of Balancing

- Breakfast consists of almond milk, sliced bananas, chia seeds, and a dusting of almonds added to overnight oats.
- Brown rice with stir-fried vegetables and chickpeas for lunch.
- Snack: Hummus-topped carrot and celery sticks
- Dinner is marinara sauce and zucchini noodles paired with lean turkey meatballs.

Day 3: Nutritious and Powerful

- Smoothie for breakfast that includes almond milk, banana, protein powder, spinach, and almond butter.
- Lunch would be a quinoa dish topped with salsa, roasted sweet potatoes, avocado, and black beans.
- A handful of mixed nuts as a snack
- Dinner is tofu and veggie skewers grilled with a side salad.

Day 4: Snacking Pleasures

- For breakfast, try these whole-grain pancakes topped with berries and Greek yogurt.
- Lunch would be whole grain rolls and lentil soup.
- Snack: Peanut butter-topped apples
- The supper is brown rice, broccoli, and bell peppers stir-fried with shrimp.

Day 5: Fulfilling Nutrition

- Avocado toast for breakfast, along with poached eggs and a dash of chili flakes
- Lunch consists of a wrap with turkey and avocado and a side salad.
- Snack: pineapple pieces mixed with cottage cheese
- Steamed asparagus and baked chicken breast with quinoa for dinner

Day 6: Complete Relishment

- Breakfast consists of a Greek yogurt parfait topped with mixed berries, granola, and maple syrup.
- Lunch is a whole wheat wrap with grilled veggies and feta cheese.
- Trail mix with nuts and dried fruits as a snack
- Supper is a brown rice stir-fried with vegetables and tofu.

Day 7: Variety in Cuisine

- Breakfast consists of whole grain bread and scrambled egg whites with sautéed spinach.
- Lunch would be a balsamic reduction, mozzarella, tomatoes, and basil in a caprese salad.
- Rice cakes with almond butter for a snack
  The supper will be roasted Brussels sprouts and baked cod with quinoa.

Delectable Recipes to Increase Metabolism

Embarking on a journey to kickstart your metabolism doesn't mean sacrificing flavor. These five mouthwatering recipes are not only delicious but also designed to ignite your metabolic fire. Feel free to savor each dish while fueling your body's energy and vitality.

1. Protein-Packed Breakfast Burrito

Ingredients:

- 2 whole grain tortillas
- 4 large eggs, scrambled
- 1 cup black beans, drained and rinsed
- 1/2 avocado, sliced
- 1/4 cup diced tomatoes
- 1/4 cup shredded cheddar cheese
- Salt, pepper, and your favorite hot sauce to taste

Instructions:

- Use a microwave or a dry skillet to reheat the tortillas.
- Scrambled eggs, black beans, sliced tomatoes, avocado slices, and shredded cheese should all be layered within each tortilla.
- Add spicy sauce, salt, and pepper for seasoning.
- After rolling the tortillas into burritos, enjoy your high-protein breakfast.

2. Quinoa and Roasted Veggie Salad

Ingredients:

- 1 cup cooked quinoa
- 1 cup mixed roasted vegetables (such as bell peppers, zucchini, and carrots)

- 1/4 cup crumbled feta cheese
- 2 tablespoons chopped fresh herbs (e.g., parsley, basil, or mint)
- Lemon vinaigrette (lemon juice, olive oil, garlic, salt, and pepper)

Instructions:

- In a bowl, mix the cooked quinoa with the roasted veggies.
- Mix in chopped herbs and crumbled feta cheese.
- Mix well after drizzling with lemon vinaigrette.
- Serve as a nutrient-dense, revitalizing salad.

3. Grilled Chicken and Vegetable Skewers

Ingredients:

- 2 boneless, skinless chicken breasts, cut into cubes
- Assorted vegetables (bell peppers, onions, zucchini, cherry tomatoes)
- Olive oil
- Lemon juice
- Garlic powder, oregano, salt, and pepper to taste

Instructions:

- Set the grill's temperature to medium-high.
- Vegetables and cubed chicken are threaded onto skewers.

- After adding a drizzle of lemon juice and olive oil, season with salt, pepper, oregano, and garlic powder.
- Turn the skewers regularly while grilling to ensure the veggies are soft and gently browned and the chicken is cooked thoroughly.
- Savor these tasty skewers as a high-protein dinner.

4. Spicy Chickpea Stir-Fry

Ingredients:

- 1 can chickpeas, drained and rinsed
- Assorted stir-fry vegetables (bell peppers, broccoli, snap peas)
- 2 tablespoons soy sauce
- 1 tablespoon sriracha sauce (adjust to taste)
- 1 teaspoon sesame oil
- 1 teaspoon grated fresh ginger
- 2 cloves garlic, minced
- Sesame seeds for garnish
- Cooked brown rice or quinoa

Instructions:

- Combine the sesame oil, ginger, garlic, sriracha, and soy sauce in a bowl.
- After preheating a pan to medium-high temperature, add the veggies and chickpeas.

- After adding the sauce to the chickpea and vegetable combination, stir-fry it until it is well-cooked and covered with sauce.
- Top with cooked quinoa or brown rice and garnish with sesame seeds.

5. Berry Protein Smoothie Bowl

Ingredients:

- 1 cup mixed berries (strawberries, blueberries, raspberries)
- 1 scoop protein powder (your choice of flavor)
- 1/2 banana
- 1/2 cup unsweetened almond milk
- Toppings: sliced banana, granola, chia seeds, shredded coconut

Instructions:

- Puree the mixed berries, almond milk, protein powder, and half of the banana till smooth.
- Transfer the blended drink to a bowl.
- For extra texture and taste, sprinkle shredded coconut, granola, chia seeds, and banana slices over top.
- Savor your smoothie bowl, which will feed and speed up your metabolism.

Week 2: Putting out the flames

Day 1: Invigorating Start

- Breakfast consists of almond milk, spinach, banana, protein powder, and smoothie.
- Lunch consists of grilled chicken salad tossed with cucumbers, cherry tomatoes, mixed greens, and lemon vinaigrette.
- Snack: Hummus-topped carrot sticks
- Supper is baked fish over quinoa and roasted Brussels sprouts.

Day 2: Consuming a Balanced Diet

- Greek yogurt parfait for breakfast, topped with granola, mixed berries, and honey drizzled over.
- Brown rice with stir-fried vegetables and lentils for lunch.
- A handful of almonds as a snack
- Dinner is whole-grain bread served with grilled veggies and tofu kebabs.

Day 3: Power of Protein

- Breakfast consists of whole grain bread and scrambled eggs with sautéed spinach.
- Lunch would be mixed greens with a turkey and avocado wrap.
- Snack: Peach slices with cottage cheese

- The supper is bell peppers filled with quinoa and a side salad.

Day 4: Complete Relishment

- For breakfast, try whole-grain pancakes topped with a dollop of Greek yogurt and mixed berries.
- Lunch is a salad of chickpeas dressed with feta cheese, chopped veggies, and balsamic vinaigrette.
- Snack: Almond butter on rice cakes
- Dinner: steamed broccoli and baked chicken breast with sweet potato mash

Day 5: Delighting in Variety

- Poached eggs on avocado toast with a dash of red pepper flakes for breakfast.
- Lunch consists of roasted chickpeas, spinach, and quinoa salad with tahini dressing.
- Snack: Peanut butter-topped apples
- Dinner is quinoa on the side and grilled fish with asparagus.

Day 6: Bright Combination

- Breakfast consists of a smoothie bowl with mixed berries, bananas, granola, and chia seeds.
- Lunch would be a fresh mozzarella, tomato, basil, and balsamic sauce caprese salad.
- Trail mix with almonds and dried fruits for a snack

- The supper will be brown rice and stir-fried shrimp with mixed veggies.

Day 7: Tasting Adventures

- Breakfast consists of chia seeds, almond milk, sliced banana, and a handful of almonds added to overnight oats.
- Lunch would be a quinoa dish with avocado, salsa, black beans, and lime dressing.
- Snack: Berries and Greek yogurt with a touch of maple syrup
- Dinner is stir-fried veggies and tofu served with whole-grain noodles.

Nutrient-Rich and Satisfying Recipes

1. Protein-Packed Quinoa Bowl

Ingredients:

- 1 cup cooked quinoa
- 4 oz grilled chicken breast, sliced
- 1 cup mixed vegetables (e.g., broccoli, bell peppers, carrots)
- 1/4 avocado, sliced
- 2 tablespoons balsamic vinaigrette

Instructions:

- Follow the directions on the box to prepare the quinoa.
- Slice the chicken breast once it has been cooked through on the grill or stove.

- Tenderize the mixed veggies by steaming or sautéing them.
- Arrange the cooked quinoa, chopped chicken, mixed veggies, avocado slices, and balsamic vinaigrette in a bowl.

Nutrition Information (approximate per serving):

- Calories: 410
- Protein: 34g
- Carbohydrates: 43g
- Fat: 16g
- Fiber: 8g

2. Mediterranean Chickpea Salad

Ingredients:

- 1 can chickpeas, drained and rinsed
- 1 cup diced cucumber
- 1 cup diced tomatoes
- 1/4 cup diced red onion
- 1/4 cup crumbled feta cheese
- 2 tablespoons olive oil
- 1 tablespoon lemon juice
- Fresh parsley, chopped

Instructions:

- Chickpeas, chopped tomatoes, diced cucumber, diced red onion, and crumbled feta cheese should all be combined in a big bowl.
- Pour lemon juice and olive oil over the mixture and toss to blend.
- Add fresh parsley as a garnish.

Nutrition Information (approximate per serving):

- Calories: 383
- Protein: 15g
- Carbohydrates: 46g
- Fat: 25g
- Fiber: 14g

3. Grilled Salmon with Quinoa and Asparagus

Ingredients:

- 6 oz grilled salmon fillet
- 1/2 cup cooked quinoa
- 1 cup steamed asparagus
- Lemon zest and juice
- Fresh dill, chopped

Instructions:

- The salmon fillet should be cooked to flaky perfection over a grill or stove.
- Follow the directions on the box to prepare the quinoa.
- Roast or steam the asparagus until it becomes soft.
- Transfer the cooked quinoa to a platter, add the grilled salmon on top, arrange the asparagus, and garnish with fresh dill, lemon juice, and zest.

Nutrition Information (approximate per serving):

- Calories: 405
- Protein: 38g
- Carbohydrates: 26g
- Fat: 24g
- Fiber: 8g

4. Berry and Almond Butter Smoothie

Ingredients:

- 1 cup mixed berries (e.g., strawberries, blueberries, raspberries)
- 1 scoop protein powder (whey or plant-based)
- 1 tablespoon almond butter
- 1 cup unsweetened almond milk,
- Ice cubes

Instructions:

- Blend mixed berries, ice cubes, almond butter, protein powder, and almond milk in a blender.
- Blend till creamy and smooth.
- Pour into a glass and start sipping right away.

Nutrition Information (approximate per serving):

- Calories: 322,
- Protein: 22g
- Carbohydrates: 25g
- Fat: 14g
- Fiber: 7g

5. Greek Yogurt Parfait

Ingredients:

- 1 cup Greek yogurt (non-fat or low-fat)
- 1/2 cup granola (opt for low-sugar)
- 1/2 cup mixed berries,
- 1 tablespoon honey

Instructions:

- Arrange Greek yogurt, granola, and mixed berries in a glass or dish.
- Pour some honey on top.

Nutrition Information (approximate per serving):

- Calories: 353
- Protein: 24g
- Carbohydrates: 53g
- Fat: 9g
- Fiber: 8g

Week 3: Keeping the Fire Guessing

Day 1: Exciting Beginning

- Breakfast consists of whole grain bread and scrambled eggs with sautéed spinach.
- Lunch would be a salad of quinoa, black beans, mixed veggies, and lime vinaigrette.
- Greek yogurt with almonds makes a healthy snack.
- Dinner is a salad on the side and a grilled turkey burger with sweet potato fries.

Day 2: Harmonious Pleasures

- Breakfast consists of a smoothie made of mixed berries, almond milk, protein powder, and chia seeds.
- Lunch consists of a grilled veggie wrap with carrot sticks on the side and hummus.
- Snack: Almond butter on sliced apples

- The supper will be baked salmon over quinoa and steamed broccoli.

Day 3: Savoury Combination

- Poached eggs on avocado toast with a dash of red pepper flakes for breakfast.
- Lunch is a dish of roasted vegetables and chickpeas with tahini dressing.
- Snack: Peach slices with cottage cheese
- The supper is brown rice and stir-fried tofu with mixed veggies.

Day 4: Complete Relishment

- Greek yogurt parfait for breakfast, topped with granola, mixed berries, and honey drizzled over.
- Lunch consists of a quinoa side dish and a spinach and feta-stuffed chicken breast.
- Trail mix with almonds and dried fruits for a snack
- Dinner is whole-grain naan with a curry of lentils and vegetables.

Day 5: Tasting Adventures

- Breakfast consists of whole-grain pancakes topped with a dollop of Greek yogurt and sliced bananas.
- Lunch would be a balsamic-glazed caprese salad topped with mozzarella, tomatoes, and basil.

- Rice cakes with almond butter for a snack
- Supper is grilled shrimp skewers paired with stir-fried quinoa and vegetables.

Day 6: Variety of Nutrients

- Breakfast consists of whole grain bread and scrambled egg whites with sautéed mushrooms.
- Lunch would be mixed greens with a turkey and avocado wrap.
- A handful of mixed nuts as a snack
- Dinner is baked fish served with a side salad and roasted Brussels sprouts.

Day 7: Exuberant Sendoff

- Breakfast consists of a smoothie bowl with mixed berries and bananas, granola, and chia seeds.
- Lunch consists of a piece of whole-grain bread and lentil and vegetable soup.
- Snack: Hummus-topped carrot and celery sticks
- Dinner is grilled bell peppers packed with quinoa and vegetables.

Inventive and Tasty Recipes to Maintain Your Metabolism Alert

1. Quinoa-Stuffed Bell Peppers

Ingredients:

- 4 large bell peppers, halved and seeds removed
- 1 cup cooked quinoa
- 1 cup black beans, drained and rinsed
- 1 cup diced tomatoes
- 1/2 cup diced red onion
- 1/2 cup shredded cheddar cheese
- 1 teaspoon cumin
- Salt and pepper, to taste

Instructions:

- Turn the oven on to 375°F, or 190°C.
- In a bowl, combine the cooked quinoa, black beans, cumin, shredded cheddar cheese, diced tomatoes, red onion, and salt and pepper.
- Spoon the quinoa mixture into each side of the bell pepper.
- Place the filled peppers on a baking sheet and bake for about 25 to 30 minutes, or until the filling is cooked through and the peppers are soft.
- Serve as a tasty, nutrient-dense dinner.

Nutrition Information (approximate per serving):

- Calories: 253
- Protein: 14g

- Carbohydrates: 47g
- Fat: 6g
- Fiber: 9g

2. Spiced Chickpea and Sweet Potato Bowl

Ingredients:

- 1 cup cooked quinoa
- 1 can chickpeas, drained and rinsed
- 1 medium sweet potato, diced
- 1 teaspoon paprika
- 1/2 teaspoon cumin
- 1/2 teaspoon turmeric
- Salt and pepper, to taste
- Olive oil, for roasting
- Mixed greens, for serving

Instructions:

- Set oven temperature to 400°F, or 200°C.
- Add olive oil, paprika, cumin, turmeric, salt, and pepper to the sweet potato and chickpeas.
- Once they are brown and crispy, spread them out on a baking sheet and roast for 20 to 25 minutes.
- In bowls, arrange cooked quinoa, sweet potato, roasted chickpeas, and mixed greens.

- Pour on your favorite sauce or dressing.

Nutrition Information (approximate per serving):

- Calories: 353
- Protein: 15g
- Carbohydrates: 68g
- Fat: 9g
- Fiber: 13g

3. Thai-inspired Coconut Curry Bowl

Ingredients:

- 1 cup cooked brown rice
- 1 cup mixed vegetables (bell peppers, carrots, snap peas)
- 1/2 cup diced tofu or cooked chicken
- 1/2 cup light coconut milk
- 1 tablespoon red curry paste
- 1 tablespoon soy sauce
- Fresh cilantro and lime wedges, for garnish

Instructions:

- Cooked mixed veggies and cubed chicken or tofu are sautéed in a skillet.
- In a bowl, whisk together coconut milk, soy sauce, and red curry paste.

- After adding the sauce to the cooked ingredients, let it boil for a little while.
- Add lime wedges and cilantro as garnish and serve over cooked brown rice.

Nutrition Information (approximate per serving):

- Calories: 320
- Protein: 13g
- Carbohydrates: 44g
- Fat: 12g
- Fiber: 8g

4. Zucchini Noodle Stir-Fry

Ingredients:

- 2 medium zucchinis, spiralized into noodles
- 1 cup cooked shrimp or tofu cubes
- 1 cup sliced bell peppers
- 1/2 cup sliced carrots
- 2 tablespoons low-sodium soy sauce
- 1 tablespoon sesame oil
- 1 teaspoon grated ginger
- 2 cloves garlic, minced
- Sesame seeds, for garnish

Instructions:

- In a wok or big pan, heat the sesame oil over medium-high heat.
- Minced garlic and grated ginger are quickly sautéed.
- Stir-fry the carrots and bell pepper slices for a few minutes.
- Add cooked shrimp or tofu and zucchini noodles; simmer for an additional two to three minutes.
- Pour in some low-sodium soy sauce and mix well.
- Serve hot with sesame seeds on top.

Nutrition Information (approximate per serving):

- Calories: 253
- Protein: 24g
- Carbohydrates: 22g
- Fat: 15g
- Fiber: 8g

5. Berry Quinoa Breakfast Bowl

Ingredients:

- 1 cup cooked quinoa
- 1/2 cup mixed berries (strawberries, blueberries, raspberries)
- 1 tablespoon almond butter
- 1 tablespoon chia seeds

- 1 tablespoon honey
- Splash of almond milk (optional)

Instructions:

- In a bowl, arrange the cooked quinoa and the mixed berries.
- Pour honey and nut butter over the blend.
- Add a few chia seeds for texture.
- If desired, add a small amount of almond milk.

Nutrition Information (approximate per serving):

- Calories: 306
- Protein: 15g
- Carbohydrates: 48g
- Fat: 9g
- Fiber: 7g

Week 4: Maximizing the Confusion

Day 1: Reviving Beginning

- Greek yogurt parfait for breakfast, topped with granola, mixed berries, and honey drizzled over.
- Lunch consists of grilled chicken salad dressed with a mild vinaigrette, cucumber, cherry tomatoes, and mixed greens.
- Snack: Hummus-topped baby carrots
- Dinner is quinoa, roasted Brussels sprouts, and baked salmon.

Day 2: Balanced Variety

- Breakfast consists of whole grain bread and scrambled eggs with sautéed spinach.
- Brown rice with stir-fried vegetables and lentils for lunch.
- A handful of almonds as a snack
- The supper is quinoa and stir-fried tofu with mixed veggies.

Day 3:

- Greek yogurt with mixed berries and whole grain pancakes for breakfast, a la Flavor Fusion
- Lunch is a roasted veggie and chickpea wrap with tahini dressing.
- Snack: Almond butter on sliced apples
- Dinner is a salad on the side and a grilled turkey burger with sweet potato fries.

Day 4: Complete Relishment

- Breakfast consists of a smoothie made of mixed berries, almond milk, protein powder, and chia seeds.
- Lunch would be a balsamic-glazed caprese salad topped with mozzarella, tomatoes, and basil.
- Snack: Peanut butter-topped rice cakes
- Dinner consists of lean ground turkey, spaghetti squash with marinara sauce, and steamed broccoli.

Day 5: Worldwide Tastes

- Poached eggs on avocado toast with a dash of red pepper flakes for breakfast.
- Lunch is a dish of quinoa and black beans with mixed veggies and cilantro-lime vinaigrette.
- Snack: A handful of mixed almonds and Greek yogurt
- Dinner is brown rice, steamed asparagus, and fish coated with a teriyaki glaze.

Day 6: Nutritious Decisions

- Breakfast consists of oatmeal with chopped almonds, banana slices, and honey drizzled over it.
- Lunch consists of a hummus and veggie wrap served with carrot sticks on the side.
- Trail mix with dried fruits and nuts makes a snack.
- Dinner is quinoa-topped baked chicken breast with roasted veggies on the side.

Day 7: Tasting Adventures

- Breakfast consists of whole grain bread and scrambled egg whites with sautéed mushrooms.
- Lunch would be a salad of chopped cucumbers, tomatoes, red onion, and feta cheese with a Mediterranean flair.
- Snack: Peach slices with cottage cheese

- The supper will be brown rice and stir-fried shrimp with mixed veggies.

Energizing and Filling Recipes that Increase Your Metabolism

1. Superfood Breakfast Bowl

Ingredients:

- 1/2 cup cooked quinoa
- 1/4 cup mixed berries (blueberries, raspberries, strawberries)
- 1 tablespoon chia seeds
- 1 tablespoon almond butter
- 1 tablespoon chopped nuts (e.g., almonds, walnuts)
- Splash of almond milk (optional)

Instructions:

- In a mixing dish, combine the cooked quinoa and berries.
- Sprinkle the chia seeds and chopped nuts on top.
- Drizzle with almond butter and a dash of almond milk for an extra creamy texture.

Nutrition Information (approximate per serving):

- Calories: 333
- Protein: 9g
- Carbohydrates: 44g

- Fat: 14g
- Fiber: 8g

2. Green Power Smoothie

Ingredients:

- 1 cup spinach or kale leaves
- 1/2 banana
- 1/2 cup mixed berries (blueberries, strawberries)
- 1 tablespoon chia seeds
- 1 scoop protein powder (whey or plant-based)
- 1 cup unsweetened almond milk

Instructions:

- Blend the spinach or kale leaves with almond milk until smooth.
- Combine bananas, mixed berries, chia seeds, and protein powder.
- Blend until completely integrated and enjoy a nutritious smoothie.

Nutrition Information (approximate per serving):

- Calories: 255
- Protein: 24g
- Carbohydrates: 33g
- Fat: 7g

- Fiber: 6g

3. Spicy Chickpea and Spinach Stir-Fry

Ingredients:

- 1 can chickpeas, drained and rinsed
- 2 cups fresh spinach leaves
- 1 small onion, thinly sliced
- 1 teaspoon cumin powder
- 1/2 teaspoon red chili flakes (adjust to taste)
- Salt and pepper, to taste
- Olive oil for cooking

Instructions:

- In a medium-sized pan, heat the olive oil.
- Add the sliced onion and sauté until transparent.
- Combine the chickpeas, cumin powder, red chili flakes, salt, and pepper. Sauté for several minutes.
- Add fresh spinach leaves and simmer until wilted.
- Serve as a spicy and healthful stir fry.

Nutrition Information (approximate per serving):

- Calories: 306
- Protein: 10g
- Carbohydrates: 43g
- Fat: 9g

- Fiber: 14g

4. Mediterranean Quinoa Salad

Ingredients:

- 1 cup cooked quinoa
- 1 cup cucumber, diced
- 1 cup cherry tomatoes, halved
- 1/2 cup crumbled feta cheese
- 1/4 cup chopped fresh parsley
- 2 tablespoons extra-virgin olive oil
- 1 tablespoon lemon juice
- Salt and pepper, to taste

Instructions:

- In a large bowl, combine cooked quinoa, diced cucumber, cherry tomatoes, feta cheese, and chopped parsley.
- In a small bowl, whisk together olive oil and lemon juice.
- Drizzle the dressing over the salad and toss to combine.
- Season with salt and pepper according to your taste.

Nutrition Information (approximate per serving):

- Calories: 354
- Protein: 13g
- Carbohydrates: 43g
- Fat: 17g

- Fiber: 6g

5. Thai-Inspired Grilled Chicken Salad

Ingredients:

- 4 oz grilled chicken breast, sliced
- 2 cups mixed greens (lettuce, spinach, arugula)
- 1/4 cup shredded carrots
- 1/4 cup chopped bell peppers (assorted colors)
- 2 tablespoons chopped peanuts
- Fresh cilantro leaves, for garnish
- Thai peanut dressing (store-bought or homemade)

Instructions:

- Decorate a platter with a variety of greens.
- To finish, garnish with grilled chicken slices, shredded carrots, chopped bell peppers, and peanuts that have been cut further.
- To finish off the salad, drizzle it with Thai peanut dressing.
- To provide an additional layer of flavor, garnish with fresh cilantro leaves.

Nutrition Information (approximate per serving):

- Calories: 355
- Protein: 33g
- Carbohydrates: 16g

- Fat: 24g
- Fiber: 5g

78

COMBINING PHYSICAL ACTIVITY WITH METABOLIC CONFUSION

The Partnership Between Nutrition and Exercise

A key component of reaching and maintaining optimum health is understanding the complex link between diet and exercise. When these two elements are carefully combined, they become a synergistic alliance that enhances general vitality, speeds up metabolism, and feeds physical well-being. Understanding the synergistic relationship between diet and exercise can open the door to a complete plan for achieving your health goals.

Activity: The Transformative Catalyst

Engaging in physical exercise is the trigger that starts the body's transformation process. Exercising in a variety of ways—whether it be yoga, weight training, cardio, or a combination of these—brings about a host of impressive advantages:

- Improved Metabolic Performance: Exercise increases metabolic rates, which makes it easier to burn calories and control weight. Additionally, it increases insulin sensitivity, which helps to maintain stable blood sugar levels.
- Improved Heart Health: Cardiovascular workouts, which include swimming and jogging, strengthen the heart, improve circulation, and lower the risk of heart disease.

- Increased Muscular Development: Strength training increases lean muscle mass, and promotes functional strength, which is essential for carrying out everyday tasks.

- Improved Skeletal Integrity: Weight-bearing activities that protect bone density, such as brisk walking and strength training, reduce the risk of osteoporosis.

- Enhancement of Mental Well-Being: Engaging in physical exercise triggers the body's endorphins, which are naturally occurring mood enhancers that help with stress reduction, mental clarity, and better sleep.

Eating Well: The Foundation of Performance

Exercise functions as the engine, and diet is the vital fuel that keeps it moving ahead. A diet rich in nutrients and well-balanced is essential for maximizing performance and accelerating recovery:

- Energy Optimization: A healthy diet is the cornerstone of maintaining energy levels, providing enough strength for everyday activities and exercise. Dinners that include proteins, carbs, and healthy fats provide consistent energy sources.

- Muscle Rejuvenation and Expansion: High-protein foods support the growth of new muscle tissue and help muscles recover after activity. This dynamic is essential for both enhanced performance and recovery.

- Micronutrient Boosting: Vitamins and minerals coordinate a range of biological processes, including immunological support, bone health, and energy production.

- Hydration Vitality: During physical activity, maintaining electrolyte balance, promoting joint lubrication, and regulating core body temperature all depend on keeping enough hydration.

- Post-Workout Recovery Nutrition: A well-balanced post-workout diet that includes a sensible proportion of both protein and carbs helps to restore glycogen stores and supports muscle repair.

The Synergy: A Wholesome Method

Exercise and diet work together to create a positive feedback loop. Your body needs more nutrients while you exercise, and eating meals high in nutrients provides the fuel your body needs for peak performance and recuperation. On the other hand, a well-balanced diet supports efficient exercise and increases the body's ability to adapt well to the demands of exercise.

Crucial Realizations:

- Customization: Acknowledge that every person has different requirements when it comes to diet and activity. Adjust them to fit your objectives, preferences, and way of life.

- Regular Exercise: Consistent exercise combined with a well-balanced diet leads to small but steady improvements in fitness and health.

- Professional Advice: Create individualized exercise and dietary plans by using the knowledge of certified dietitians and fitness specialists.

- Long-Term Outlook: Adopt a forward-looking perspective. The relationship between diet and exercise is a lifetime journey toward better health and well-being.

Customizing Your Exercise Program to Boost Metabolic Impact

Tailoring Your Exercise Program for the Best Metabolic Effect

Developing an exercise program that maximizes the benefits of your metabolism is a calculated move toward improving your fitness level. Exercise regimens that are in line with metabolic objectives may increase energy expenditure, speed up the burning of calories, and encourage long-term gains in general health. Here's how to modify your exercise regimen to get powerful metabolic effects:

- Adopt High-Intensity Interval Training (HIIT): Combine brief intervals of high-intensity exercise with rest intervals. In addition to burning calories during exercise, high-intensity interval training (HIIT) causes your body to continue burning calories afterward.

- Boost Strength Training: To increase muscular growth, include resistance workouts such as bodyweight exercises or weightlifting. Because muscles have an active metabolism, they continue to burn calories even while at rest.

- Make Compound Movements a Priority: Give special attention to compound workouts that work many muscle groups at once. Compared to standalone workouts, squats, deadlifts, and bench presses increase the metabolic response.

- Include Cardiovascular Work: To increase heart rate and improve cardiovascular health, do cardio exercises like cycling, swimming, or running. Cardio exercises increase metabolic efficiency and encourage calorie expenditure.

- Change Up Your Exercises: To avoid plateaus and promote metabolic adaptability, switch up your workouts. A varied program pushes the body to new limits and encourages ongoing development.

- Integrate Circuit Training: Create a circuit-style workout by combining cardio and weight training. This method increases the metabolic needs by contracting your muscles and maintaining an elevated heart rate.

- Choose Active Rest: To keep your heart rate up and your metabolism going during rest periods, try doing some light walking or dynamic stretches.

- Make Post-Workout Nutrition a Priority: After working out, eat a balanced meal high in carbs and protein. Restoring glycogen reserves and promoting muscle repair, promotes a healthy metabolism.

- Take Part in Regular Physical Activity: Move a part of your everyday routine by walking, climbing stairs, or standing up and down sometimes. All of these behaviors add up to a more active metabolism.

- Track your progress and make necessary adjustments to the intensity, length, and exercises of your workouts. Steady development guarantees sustained metabolic gains.

- Make Sure You Get Enough Rest and Recovery: Give good sleep a top priority and give your muscles enough time to heal. Inadequate sleep might impair progress and metabolic function.

- Remain Hydrated: Make sure you get enough water before, during, and after your exercises. Hydration is essential for metabolic functions.

- Speak with a Fitness Professional: Get advice from professionals in the field of fitness to develop a program that is unique to your objectives, level of fitness, and any particular health issues.

Recuperation Techniques for Best Outcomes

Using recuperation strategies strategically is essential to getting the most out of your exercise pursuits. Adopting efficient recovery techniques is crucial for encouraging muscle regeneration, reducing tiredness, and maintaining improvement, just as your exercises push your body. Through the integration of focused recuperation techniques, you can guarantee that your body stays prepared for regular and effective activity. To optimize your outcomes, use these tips for smoothly integrating rehabilitation into your daily routine:

- Make Sleep a Priority: Try to get between seven and nine hours of good sleep every night. Effective recuperation begins with restorative sleep, which promotes hormone balance, tissue repair, and brain renewal.

- Hydration Is Important: Make sure you stay well hydrated all day. Temperature control, nutrition transport, and muscular function are all aided by hydration. Before, during, and after your exercises, sip water.

- Accept Active Recovery: On your days off, take part in low-impact, mild exercise like yoga, strolling, or light stretching. Active recuperation improves flexibility, reduces pain in the muscles, and increases blood flow.

- Fuel Your Recovery: Have a post-workout meal that is well-balanced and high in carbs and protein. This promotes effective recovery by nourishing muscle regeneration and assisting in the replenishment of glycogen storage.

- Apply Self-Myofascial Alleviate: Use massage techniques or foam rolling to release tension in tense muscles. This method promotes blood flow and facilitates the healing of muscles.

- Dynamic Stretching: As part of your pre-workout warm-up, use dynamic stretches. These stretches increase flexibility and prime muscles for movement. To improve your range of motion, use static stretches after working out.

- Take Contrast Baths or Showers: To promote circulation and lessen muscular inflammation, alternate between hot and cold water immersion. Start with warm water and end with a quick dip in the cold.

- Pay Attention to Your Body: Recognize the warning signals of overtraining, which include chronic weariness, diminished performance, and mood swings. When you need it, give yourself more time to relax.

- Accept Scheduled Rest Days: Include specified rest days in your weekly routine. These pauses allow muscles the time they need for recovery and guard against burnout.

- Develop Mindfulness and Relaxation: To reduce stress and support your mental health, try deep breathing exercises, meditation, or moderate yoga.

- Professional Advice: If you're having trouble with certain muscular problems, think about consulting with a sports massage therapist or physical therapist for customized healing therapies.

- Adopt Consistency: It is essential to practice recovery techniques regularly. Recovering consistently is a very effective way to prevent overuse injuries and improve overall function.

- Modify Your Approach: To prevent overtraining and promote continuous improvement, periodically adjust the amount and intensity of your workouts.

- Keep an Optimistic Attitude: Your recuperation process may be greatly impacted by having a positive outlook. Remain patient and acknowledge your victories as you strive toward your fitness objectives.

- Track Your Progress: Keep tabs on your physical and rehabilitation progress. This aids in determining the tactics that work best for the demands of your body.

EXTENDED-TERM INTEGRATION OF LIFESTYLE

Changing to a Post-Plan Sustainable Diet

When your meal plan adventure comes to an end, switching to a sustainable post-plan diet is an essential step to sustaining your gains and keeping up a healthy lifestyle. Consider this the beginning of a lifetime commitment to well-being rather than its conclusion. Here's a how-to for navigating this shift with ease and effectiveness:

- Gradual Changes: Steer clear of abrupt adjustments. Reintroduce items that were off-limits for the duration of the plan gradually while maintaining portion control. This keeps you from overindulging and enables your body to adjust to a greater variety of meals.

- Accept Food Diversity: To guarantee a well-rounded nutritional intake, make room for a range of foods. Add dairy products or appropriate substitutes, fruits, vegetables, entire grains, lean proteins, and healthy fats.

- Portion Consciousness: Keep an eye out for serving sizes to prevent overindulging. Pay attention to your body's signals of hunger and fullness so you may modify how much you eat.

- Track Your Progress: Pay attention to your weight, energy levels, and the way your body responds to certain meals. You may adjust your diet based on your fitness goals and overall well-being with the aid of this information.

- Hydration Maintenance: Make staying hydrated a top priority by consuming enough water throughout the day. Maintaining enough hydration promotes healthy metabolism, digestion, and general energy.

- Mindful Eating Practices: Practice mindful eating by taking your time, enjoying every mouthful, and paying attention to your body's cues about whether it's hungry or full.

- Continue Regular Exercise: To maintain your muscle mass, metabolic rate, and overall health, stick to your prescribed exercise regimen. Engaging in physical exercise also improves your mood and helps you handle stress.

- Create Well-Balanced Meals: Plan your meals to include a healthy balance of protein, healthy fats, carbs, and plenty of veggies. This ensures that you get the nourishment you need.

- Moderate Indulgences: Treating yourself once in a while is OK, but only in moderation. This helps to have a pleasant connection with food and avoids emotions of lack.

- Pay Attention to Your Body: Pay attention to how your body reacts to various meals. Take note of any pain or changes in your energy level and adjust your selections appropriately.

- Patience and Flexibility: Keep in mind that each person's path is unique. Be patient with yourself and don't worry about sporadic deviations. Retaining both consistency and flexibility is crucial.

- Accept Long-Term Well-Being: Change your focus from immediate objectives to long-term health. Accept the path of taking care of your health and mind in the years to come.

Maintaining the Metabolic Fire for Eternity

Long-term health and vigor are largely dependent on sustaining a robust metabolism. Your dedication to well-being is a lifelong commitment, not just a plan for the near future. Here's how to make sure that when you set out on a path to vigorous, lifetime health, the metabolic fire never goes out:

- Develop Steadfastness: A robust metabolism is built on steadfastness. Continue to be committed to regular exercise, a well-balanced diet, and the healthy habits you've adopted along the road.
- Adopt Sustainable Nutrition: Give up strict diets and adopt a long-term eating schedule that nourishes your body with a variety of nutritious foods. Give dietary variety, moderation, and nutritional richness top priority.
- Champion Protein Intake: To support muscle building and maintenance, include lean protein throughout your meals. Foods high in protein also increase the thermic effect, which increases the amount of calories used up during digestion.

- Resistance Training: Include resistance training in your exercise routine. Strength training helps to maintain muscle mass, which ensures an active metabolism as people age.

- Remain Active: Steer clear of prolonged periods of inactivity. Move throughout the day; take short walks, stretch, or indulge in other gentle exercises to keep your metabolism going.

- Effectively Handle Stress: Chronic stress might affect the metabolism. Use techniques for relieving stress, such as yoga, meditation, or deep breathing, to keep your hormones in balance.

- Make Sleep a Priority: Getting a good night's sleep is essential for healthy metabolism. Aim for seven to nine hours of restorative sleep per night to promote hormonal balance and energy management.

- Drink enough water to be well-hydrated. Hydration is your ally. Water is essential for several metabolic functions, such as nutrition transport, and digestion.

- Select Entire Grains: Make your choice from whole grains including whole wheat, quinoa, and brown rice. They help regulate metabolism, prevent blood sugar surges, and provide prolonged energy.

- Accept Fiber-Rich Options: Include foods high in fiber in your diet, such as fruits, vegetables, and legumes. They improve blood sugar regulation, improve digestion, and promote healthy gut flora.

- Keep an Eye on Your Progress: Keep track of your fitness and health progress. You can remain in alignment and make any modifications with the support of regular evaluations.

- Utilize Intuitive Eating: Pay attention to your body's signals of hunger and satisfaction. Feed when you're hungry and stop when you're full to maintain a healthy metabolism.

- Cultivate Curiosity and Open-Mindedness: Continue expanding your knowledge of nutrition, fitness, and well-being. Welcome creative ways that connect with your objectives and lifestyle.

- Revel in the Voyage: Remember that a healthy metabolism is the outcome of lifetime activities. Accept the trip, acknowledge your successes, and relish the advantages for your overall well-being.

Observing and Modifying Your Method Over Time

It's critical to realize that tracking your progress and making necessary adjustments to your tactics over time is a critical component of achieving long-term health and well-being. Your journey is a never-ending process that needs constant assessment and modification. Here's how to successfully monitor your development and make the required adjustments to keep going forward:

- Frequent Self-Reflection: Set aside time for routine self-evaluation. Think back on your objectives, successes, and any challenges you've faced. Being self-aware helps in maintaining your alignment with your goals.

- Use Tracking Tools: Keep a record of your daily activities, meals, and feelings by using tools such as notebooks, fitness trackers, or smartphone applications. This information sheds light on trends and potential problem areas.

- Listen to Your Body: Observe how your body reacts to your daily routine. Track changes in your mood, energy, digestion, and sleep patterns. You may make course modifications based on these indications.

- Review Your Objectives: Review your objectives regularly. Are they still reachable and relevant? Adjust them as needed to reflect your changing goals and situation in life.

- Celebrate Milestones: Whether they are little successes or breakthroughs, acknowledge and honor your accomplishments. Realizing your progress gives you more willpower to keep going.

- Seek Expert Advice: For unbiased advice, consult a fitness coach, nutritionist, or healthcare professional. Their knowledge might provide insightful guidance for improving your tactics.

- Adjust to Shifts in Lifestyle: As life is ever-changing, so should your strategy. Modify your approaches to account for changes in your family, job, or other obligations.

- Try New Things and Learn: Investigate new foods, workouts, or regimens. Embrace an experimental mindset to find what suits your body and tastes the best.

- Overcome Plateaus: In the face of progress plateaus, don't be disheartened. Such phases are common. Identify likely reasons and try with modifications to revive your momentum.

- Accept Flexibility: Don't be afraid to make changes to your strategy. Things that worked well for you in the past may need to be adjusted as your body changes and your situation changes.

- Make Sustainable Behaviors Your Top Priority: Give your whole attention to long-term sustainable habits. Sustainable practices guarantee long-term development and welfare.

- Develop a Positive Attitude: Make your approach positive. Accept difficulties as opportunities for development and see changes as milestones in the right direction.

- Exercise Patience: It takes time for results to show. Remain patient and dedicated, realizing that little adjustments made consistently add up to big results.

- Reestablish Your Motivation by thinking back on the inspiration for your trip. You may rekindle your determination by reconnecting with your reasons.
- Accept Lifelong Learning: Get more knowledge about exercise, diet, and overall health. Knowing enables you to make well-informed judgments and carefully modify your strategy.

CONCLUSION

We have extensively investigated the complexities of metabolic confusion and its potential to transform our perspective on well-being throughout the trip we have undertaken. We have investigated every aspect of creating a healthy, sustainable lifestyle. We've mapped out a thorough route to holistic well-being, from solving the metabolic puzzle and realizing the critical role hormones play in regulation to creating customized diet plans and adopting an adaptive mentality.

The discovery of metabolic confusion, a novel idea that uses rotation and diversity to boost metabolism, marked the beginning of our journey. This ground-breaking method breaks through barriers, maintains advancement, and cultivates a balanced, healthy physique. We learned a great deal about hormones and their complex role in metabolic regulation, which helped us understand how our internal processes affect our general health.

As we investigated metabolic confusion's capacity to boost metabolic energy, promote fat loss, and protect lean muscle mass, its advantages for weight control were clear. The mystery surrounding macronutrients was solved, highlighting their critical function in creating balanced meals that provide our bodies with the best possible nourishment and energy. By aligning our meals with our bodies' inherent cycles and understanding the fluctuations of

96

calories and macronutrients, we created vital habits that support a healthy metabolism.

After that, we traveled through real-world terrain where we created customized rotation schedules and modified tactics to fit various lifestyles. With everything from very thorough meal planning to energizing dishes, every week provided a special set of tools for maintaining long-term health. We strengthened the foundation of our journey by including exercise, understanding the relationship between diet and fitness, and developing recuperation techniques.

However, our journey went beyond menus and cooking instructions. We explored the areas of fostering a positive atmosphere, establishing realistic objectives, and welcoming difficulties as opportunities for development. We learned the skill of maintaining the metabolic spark for life as we made the shift to a post-plan diet; this was a journey characterized by flexibility, endurance, and a never-ending quest for knowledge.

Our journey toward metabolic mastery ultimately leads us to the understanding that maintaining good health is a lifetime effort. It's a fabric made of mindful eating, regular exercise, a balanced diet, and a dynamic attitude. With the knowledge gained from metabolic confusion, we are better able to make informed decisions that will benefit our bodies, brains, and souls over the long term.

Accept this information, use it wisely, and use it to motivate you in your quest for long-term health and vitality. Remember that while you navigate the complex pathways of metabolism, your route is distinct, your advancement is noteworthy, and your legacy of lifetime well-being is something you painstakingly create with every choice you make.

BONUS

Shopping Lists for a Healthier Diet

Smart food shopping is the first step in improving your eating habits. To help you make healthful choices, here are two example shopping lists: one comprehensive enough for a week of wholesome meals, and the other specific to a plant-based diet:

Protein Sources:

- Skinless chicken breasts
- Lean ground turkey
- Fresh salmon fillets
- Greek yogurt (low-fat)
- Farm-fresh eggs

Carbohydrates:

- Whole-grain bread or wraps
- Nutrient-rich quinoa
- Fiber-packed brown rice
- Wholesome sweet potatoes
- Nutrient-dense oats

Assortment of Veggies:

- Vibrant spinach
- Cruciferous broccoli

- Colorful bell peppers
- Vitamin-rich carrots
- Versatile zucchini

Natural Fruits:

- Crisp apples
- Antioxidant-rich berries (blueberries, strawberries)
- Nutrient-loaded bananas
- Zesty citrus fruits (oranges, grapefruits)

Dairy or Dairy Alternatives:

- Nut milk (almond, soy, etc.)
- Low-fat cottage cheese

Nutritional Nuts and Seeds:

- Crunchy almonds
- Nutrient-packed chia seeds

Wholesome Fats:

- Creamy avocado
- Heart-healthy olive oil

Sample Grocery List for Plant-Powered Eating:

Plant-Based Protein:

- Versatile tofu
- Protein-rich lentils

- Versatile chickpeas
- Complete-protein quinoa
- Nutrient-packed tempeh

Carbohydrate Choices:

- Whole-grain pasta
- Fiber-packed brown rice
- Wholesome oats

Variety of Veggies:

- Robust kale
- Nurturing spinach
- Juicy tomatoes
- Colorful bell peppers
- Adaptable cauliflower

Natural Fruits:

- Satiating bananas
- Antioxidant-packed berries (strawberries, raspberries)
- Crisp apples
- Flavorful mangoes

Dairy Alternatives:

- Plant-based milk (almond, oat, etc.)

Plant-Powered Nuts and Seeds:

- Nutty walnuts
- Nutrient-rich flaxseeds

Wholesome Fats:

- Creamy avocado
- Versatile coconut oil

Tips:

- Customize these lists to fit your nutritional needs and dietary choices.
- To improve your dishes, think about adding a range of herbs, spices, and condiments.
- Focus on the outside aisles of the supermarket to find plant-based substitutes, lean meats, and fresh veggies.
- When possible, try to eat complete, unprocessed meals.